Generis

PUBLISHING

Comparison of imo and Humphrey field analyzer perimeters in glaucomatous eyes

Yoshihide Nakai

Title: Comparison of imo and Humphrey field analyzer perimeters in glaucomatous eyes

ISBN: 978-1-63902-864-1

Author: Yoshihide Nakai

Cover image: www.pixabay.com

Publisher: Generis Publishing
Online orders: www.generis-publishing.com
Contact email: info@generis-publishing.com

Abstract

AIM: To compare the imo perimeter, a new portable head-mounted perimeter unit that enables both eyes to be examined quickly and simultaneously, with the Humphrey field analyzer (HFA) perimeter to investigate correlations and their diagnostic ability in glaucomatous eyes.

METHODS: We tested the performance of this equipment in 128 glaucomatous eyes and 40 normal eyes. We investigated the correlations of mean deviation, pattern standard deviation, and visual field index and the sensitivity. The imo perimeter had a short measurement time, and compared with HFA, the imo perimeter showed no significant difference between each parameter and the diagnostic ability.

RESULTS: Measurements of mean deviation ($r=0.886$, $P<0.001$), pattern standard deviation ($r=0.814$, $P<0.001$), and visual field index ($r=0.871$, $P<0.001$) in both perimeters were strongly and positively correlated. The sensitivities in the imo perimeter were 80.5% for mean deviation, 81.2% for pattern standard deviation, and 80.5% in visual field index; those in the HFA were 63.3% for mean deviation, 74.5% for pattern standard deviation, and 80.5% for visual field index. Both perimeters demonstrated high diagnostic ability.

CONCLUSION: The parameters by the imo and HFA in glaucomatous eyes show strong positive correlations with favorable sensitivity, specificity, and diagnostic ability. However, the difference between imo and HFA results increases with the increase in visual field disturbance.

KEYWORDS: imo perimeter; visual field diagnosis; diagnostic validation

DOI:10.18240/ijo.2021.12.

Citation: Nakai Y, Bessho K, Shono Y, Taoka K, Nakai Y. Comparison of imo and Humphrey field analyzer perimeters in glaucomatous eyes. *Int J Ophthalmol* 2021;14(12):

INTRODUCTION

An automated visual field analyzer (perimeter) is indispensable for glaucoma diagnosis and follow-up. However, the conventional equipment is heavy, and a large amount of installation space is needed, and the examining room must be dark. For an examination, patients must sit in front of the visual field analyzer; therefore, bedside examinations are not possible. Recently, however, a head-mounted device, the imo perimeter (Crewt Medical Systems, Inc., Tokyo, Japan), has been developed to be lightweight (1.8 kg) and to be used in a brightly lit room. It can help clinicians perform visual field inspections and observe the central and peripheral visual fields of up to 30 degrees in both eyes simultaneously within a short time period (Figure 1)[1-11].

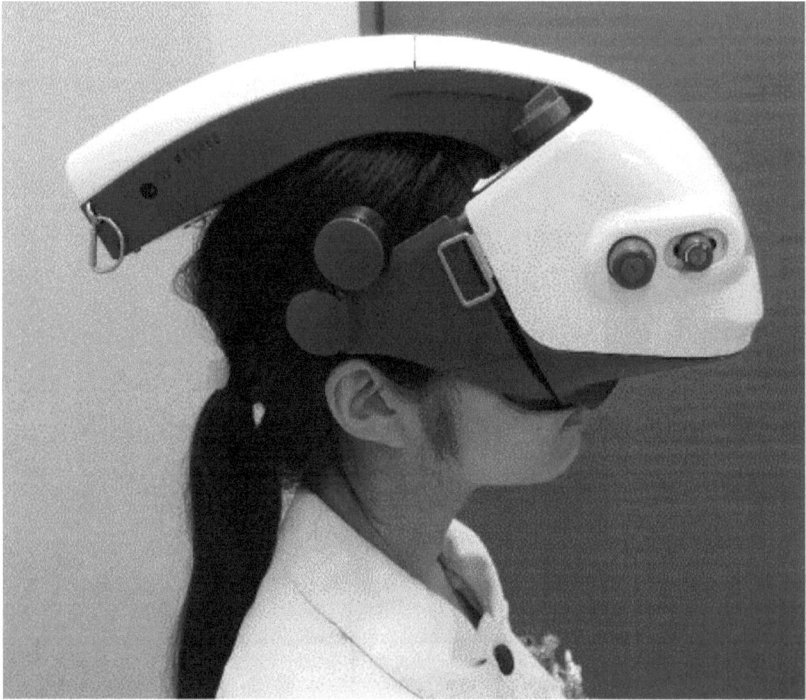

Figure 1: Head-mounted imo perimeter weighing 1.8 kg It can be used in a well-lit room, and it enables both eyes to be examined quickly and simultaneously.

We compared glaucoma detection sensitivities, diagnostic abilities in addition to the correlation of each parameter and examination time of the Humphrey field analyzer (HFA; Humphrey Instruments, Dublin, CA, USA), which is currently in wide use, with those of imo perimeters.

With the imo perimeter, the left and right pupils are monitored individually with a near-infrared camera for fixation disparity, which reduces the examination time (Figure 2). In addition, with the imo perimeter, a transmissive liquid crystal display at full high-definition resolution and a high-brightness light-emitting diode backlight are used in the same conditions as those of the HFA perimeter. Furthermore, targets are shown to the left and right eyes of subjects separately but simultaneously by independent left and right optical systems. In the visual field test, the fixed target is visually fused, and patients fixate on the target with both eyes open (Figure 3).

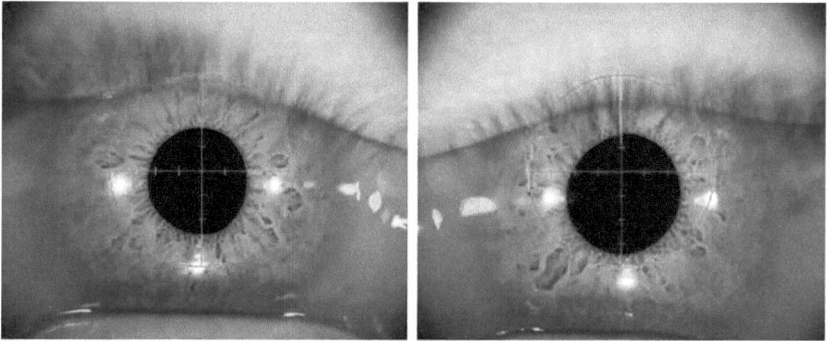

Figure 2: Simultaneous monitoring of binocular fixation by imo perimeter, with automatic tracking correction (from side to side and up and down), and pupil diameter measurement.

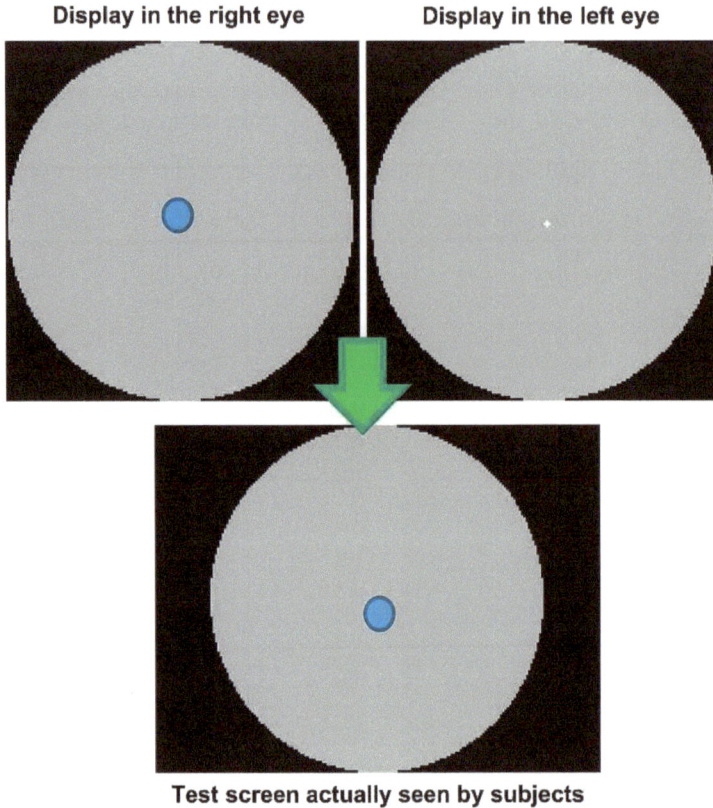

Display in the right eye　　　**Display in the left eye**

Test screen actually seen by subjects

Figure 3: The test target was presented randomly to either eye under a nonocclusion condition, and the patient was not aware of which eye was being tested.

The imo perimeter has a mode of 24 plus (78 test points) to which a 10-2 visual field is added (so that it is partially like the HFA perimeter with its visual fields of 30-2, 24-2, and 10-2), as well as a mode of 24 plus 1 (36 points), in which the points are preferentially focused on sites in which disease is likely to occur. To examine the correlation of the measurements made with the HFA and imo perimeters for mild to severe glaucoma, we used a 30-2 examination program (widely used in glaucoma diagnosis), in which a 30-degree visual field was measured with intervals of 6 degrees.

SUBJECTS AND METHODS

Ethical Approval

This study was conducted in compliance with the tenets of the Helsinki Declaration, and all participants provided written informed consent.

Visual field tests were performed with both the HFA and imo perimeters on the same day for each patient on 128 eyes of 64 patients with glaucoma and 40 normal eyes of 20 healthy people, all of whom were examined at the Tokai Eye Clinic, Tsu, Japan, between October 2018 and February 2019. Patients with glaucoma who completely understood the contents of the visual field tests and demonstrated good visual fixation in testing were selected.

Using Pearson's correlation coefficient, we compared the parameters—the mean deviation and defect (MD), the pattern standard deviation (PSD), and the visual field index (VFI)—as measured by both the HFA and imo perimeters. We calculated the detection sensitivity by using Bland–Altman analysis, the diagnostic ability by the area under the receiver operating characteristic curve (AUC), and, with the *t* test, the examination time.

Background of Patients with Glaucoma

The participants with glaucoma had a spherical equivalent of -6 D to +3 D, astigmatism of ±2.5 D, and best-corrected visual acuity (logMAR) of 0.2 to

0.08 they had not undergone eye surgery in the past and had no eye disease except glaucoma. The patients were 18 to 72 years of age, with an average age of 59.5±13.5y; 25 were men, and 39 were women (Table 1).

Table 1 Characteristics of the participants in the study

Parameters	Normal, 20 cases (40 eyes)	Glaucoma, 64 cases (128 eyes)
Age (y)		
Mean±SD	54.8±13.2	59.5±13.5
Range	(20-67)	(18-72)
Gender, *n* (%)		
Female	12 (60)	39 (61)
Male	8 (40)	25 (39)
Spherical equivalent (D)		
Mean±SD	-1.75±1.2	-2.51±2.0
Range	-5.5 to 2.5	-6 to 3
Best-corrected visual acuity (log MAR),		
Mean±SD	0.13±0.06	0.09±0.06
Range	0.2 to 0.01	0.2 to 0.08
Cylindric value (D)		
Mean±SD	1.1±0.041	1.5±0.75
Range	-2 to 2.8	-2.5 to 2.5
History of intraocular surgery	-	-
Ocular disease other than glaucoma	-	-

RESULTS

In the 40 normal eyes, the mean examination times were 12±1.4min with the HFA perimeter and 8.3±1.8min with the imo perimeter (*P*<0.001). In the 128 glaucomatous eyes, the mean examination times were 16.2±2.5min with the HFA perimeter and 12.0±2.5min with the imo perimeter (*P*<0.001). Thus the examinations of both the normal eyes and the eyes with glaucoma were performed in a significantly short time (*P*<0.001; Table 2).

Table 2 Examination time of imo and HFA perimeters

mean±SD

Condition of eye	*n*	imo perimeter	HFA perimeter	imo-HFA Comparison	*P*
Glaucomatous	128	12±2.5	16.2±2.5	-4.2±2.2	<0.001
Normal	40	8.3±1.8	12±1.4	-3.8±2.5	<0.001

HFA: Humphrey field analyzer, SD: Standard deviation.

Pearson's correlation coefficients with the HFA and imo perimeters in the 128 eyes with glaucoma were 0.886 (*P*<0.001) for MD, 0.814 (*P*<0.001) for PSD, and 0.871 (*P*<0.001) for VFI; strong correlations were thus noted. In the 40 normal eyes, the correlation coefficients were 0.248 (*P*<0.124) for MD, 0.111 (*P*<0.496) for PSD, and 0.028 (*P*<0.864) for VFI (Figure 4).

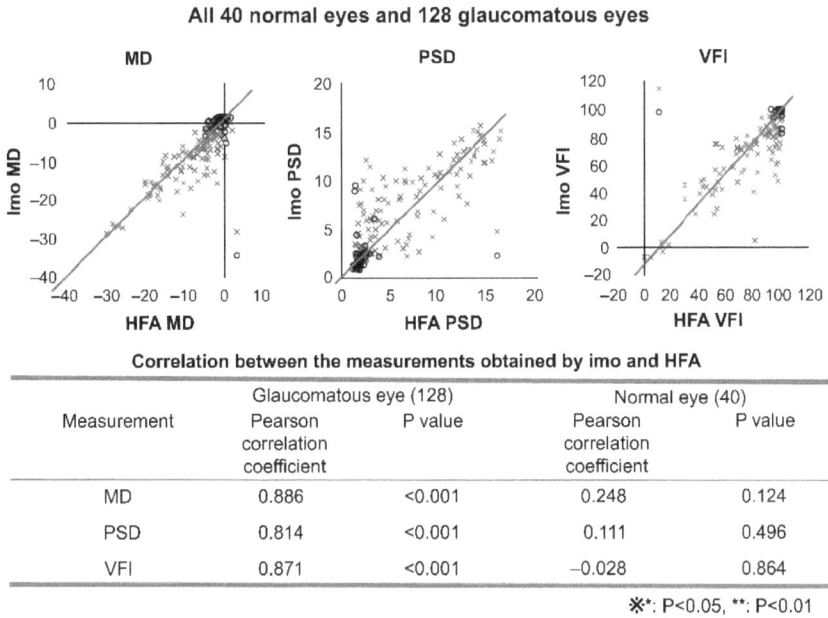

All 40 normal eyes and 128 glaucomatous eyes

Correlation between the measurements obtained by imo and HFA

Measurement	Glaucomatous eye (128)		Normal eye (40)	
	Pearson correlation coefficient	P value	Pearson correlation coefficient	P value
MD	0.886	<0.001	0.248	0.124
PSD	0.814	<0.001	0.111	0.496
VFI	0.871	<0.001	−0.028	0.864

※*: P<0.05, **: P<0.01

Figure 4: In 128 glaucomatous eyes, the imo perimeter and the HFA perimeter's measurements of MD (r=0.886, P<0.001), PSD (r=0.814, P<0.001), and VFI (r=0.871, P<0.001) were strongly and positively correlated.

To compare the MD, PSD, and VFI measured by both the perimeters, we performed the Bland–Altman analysis because even if those parameters of the HFA and imo perimeters were correlated, we suspected a difference would reflect a worse rate of glaucoma. Figure 5 illustrates the results of a comparison of the visual field findings of the HFA and imo perimeters in patients 1, 2, 3, and 4. Patient 1, in whom glaucoma was mild, showed no difference in parameters, whereas patients 2, 3 and 4, in whom the glaucoma was advanced, did show differences. The results of the Bland–Altman analysis are shown in Figure 6, in which the vertical axis reflects the difference between the imo and HFA perimeters and the horizontal axis shows the average values of the HFA and imo perimeters. The distribution was fan-shaped, whereby the worse the glaucoma was (horizontal axis), the greater was the difference in results between the imo and HFA perimeters. This finding reflects a proportional error.

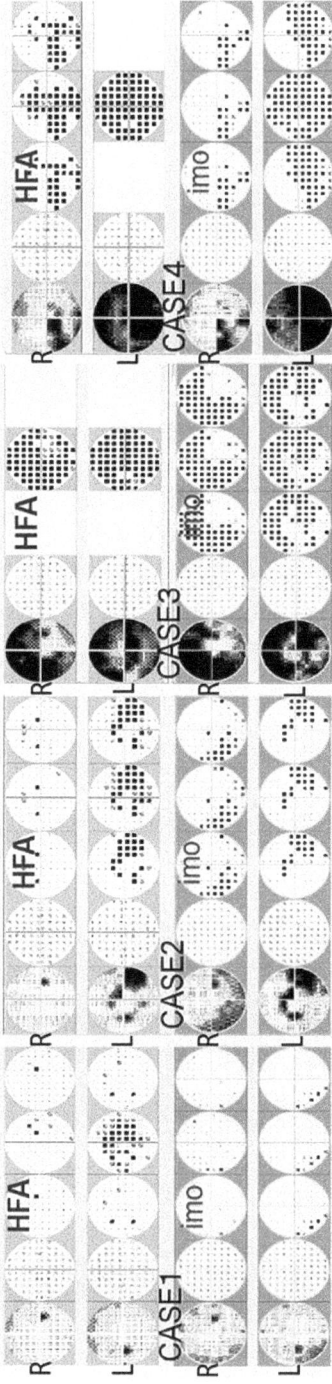

Figure 5: Displays of the visual field by the HFA and imo perimeters In case 1 (mild glaucoma), there was no difference in the displays; in case 2, 3 and 4 (advanced glaucoma), however, the differences were obvious.

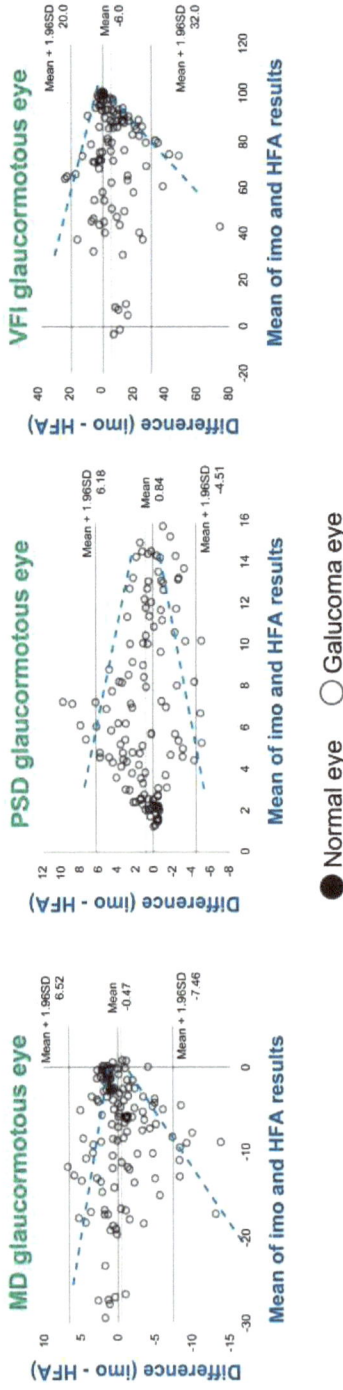

Figure 6: Bland–Altman analysis was used to compare MD, PSD, and VFI measurements by the HFA perimeter and the imo perimeter. For glaucoma eye a proportional error was observed The results show the fan-shaped distribution, where the worse is the glaucoma (horizontal axis), the greater is the difference between imo and HFA results.

The diagnostic ability of both perimeters was examined with AUC (Figure 7). The vertical axis represents sensitivity, and the horizontal axis represents specificity. For MD, the AUCs were 0.911 for the imo perimeter and 0.819 for the HFA perimeter; for PSD, they were 0.885 for the imo perimeter and 0.890 for the HFA perimeter; and for VFI, they were 0.882 for the imo perimeter and 0.872 for the HFA perimeter. Both the imo and HFA perimeters demonstrated high diagnostic ability, and no significant difference in diagnostic ability was noted between them.

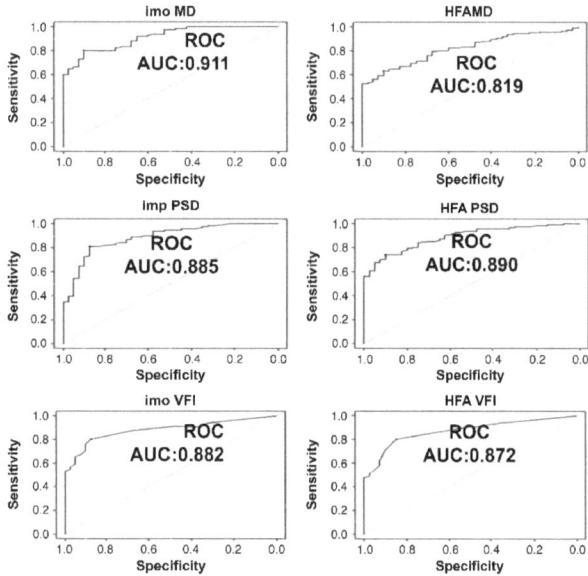

Ability of imo and HFA diagnosing glaucoma

Measurement	Device	AUC	Lower limit	Upper limit	P value*1	Sensitivity	Specificity	Cut-off value	P value*2
MD	imo	0.911	0.867	0.955	<0.001	80.5%	90.0%	Below-1.67, diagnosed with glaucoma	0.002**
	HFA	0.819	0.756	0.883	<0.001	63.3%	90.0%	Below-3.37, diagnosed with glaucoma	
PSD	imo	0.885	0.828	0.941	<0.001	81.2%	87.5%	2.74 or higher, diagnosed with glaucoma	0.876
	HFA	0.890	0.840	0.939	<0.001	74.2%	90.0%	2.37 or higher, diagnosed with glaucoma	
VFI	imo	0.882	0.831	0.933	<0.001	80.5%	87.5%	Below-1.67, diagnosed with glaucoma	0.717
	HFA	0.872	0.817	0.926	<0.001	80.5%	85.0%	Below-1.67, diagnosed with glaucoma	

Figure 7: The vertical axis represents sensitivity, and the horizontal axis represents specificity　The diagnostic abilities of both the HFA and the imo perimeters were significant; AUC was 0.8 or greater in the MD, PSD, and VFI measurements, and the maximum value of the AUC was 0.911 for the MD measurement by the imo perimeter.

DISCUSSION

In addition to 30-2, 24-2, and 10-2 perimetry inspection modes, which the HFA perimeter has, the imo perimeter has a mode termed "24 plus" (78 test points). This mode consists of some of the test points of 10-2 added to those of 24-2(36 test points), in which test points are preferentially arranged at sites of the 24 plus mode in which disease is likely to occur. An algorithm termed "AIZE-Rapid" (Crewt Medical Systems) can be used to further shorten inspection time. The imo perimeter is highly reliable because it has two independent optical systems that can both perform a visual field examination with both the patient's eyes open and perform eye tracking of the pupil.

In this study, 128 eyes of 64 glaucoma patients and 40 eyes of 20 healthy people were examined with the 30-2 mode, which is widely currently used in glaucoma testing. The current basic measurement of static visual field consists of examining approximately 70 measurements points within the central 30 degrees with intervals of 6 degrees, as indicated by the HFA perimeter 30-2 mode. The arrangement of the grid-like measurement points with intervals of 6 degrees has poor sensitivity for early glaucoma detection and macular disease; therefore, the use of an additional macular mode such as 10-2 is recommended.

The purpose of this study was to investigate the correlation between imo and HFA perimeter and the reliability of imo perimeter. Therefore, in many cases, abnormalities appeared early within 30 degrees of the visual field center. In 30-2, comparison of measurement time of two perimeters, the correlation of each parameter, Bland–Altman analysis, and diagnostic ability with AUC were examined.

In the comparison between the widely used HFA and the Octopus perimeters[12] and in comparison with the KOWA AP-7000 perimeter[13] reported strong correlations. With regard to the effect of different arrangements, these investigators reported that there was no substantial difference between the 30-2 and 24-2 modes to the HFA perimeter[14-15]. As our objective was to examine the correlation between the imo and HFA perimeters and the reliability of the imo perimeter, we compared the measurement times of both perimeters by using the 30-2 mode. This is the mode in which abnormalities caused by many diseases are expressed earliest within the central 30 degrees of the visual field. We checked the correlation of each parameter, performed a Bland–Altman analysis, and used the AUC to examine the glaucoma diagnostic ability of both perimeters.

Khoury *et al*[14] compared the examination times of the HFA with 24-2 and 30-2 modes, demonstrating an average of 10min and 24 seconds with the 24-2 mode and an average of 14min and 24 seconds with the 30-2 mode. Our examinations of 128 glaucomatous eyes and 40 normal eyes were significantly shorter with the imo perimeter than with the HFA perimeter: shorter by 4.2min for glaucomatous eyes and by 3.8min for normal eyes (Table 2). Because the imo perimeter is capable of measuring both eyes simultaneously in a brightly lit room, the burden on patients was reduced. It is thought that the examination time with the imo perimeter is shorter because it individually monitors the fixation of the left and right pupils and automatically corrects fixation disparity and because the AIZE-Rapid algorithm further speeds up examination.

Pearson's correlation coefficients of MD, PSD, and VFI were 0.886, 0.814, and 0.871 (all $P<0.001$), respectively, and the correlations were significantly positive (Figure 4). In normal eyes, the reason that the MD, PSD, and VFI were 0.248, 0.111, and 0.028 and were lower than those in glaucomatous eyes was probably because the parameter values of normal eyes was dense. Even though there was a positive correlation between the two perimeters, we performed a Bland–Altman analysis to examine whether there was any difference as a result of the progression of glaucoma. The analysis showed that the difference between the imo and HFA perimeters tended to increase as glaucoma progressed, and a proportional error was observed in MD, PSD, and VFI in all cases (Figure 5). Thus caution is required in the determinations of these parameters because the difference between results obtained with the imo and HFA perimeters increases as the visual field disturbance progresses. This demonstrates that the measurements obtained from the imo may indicate a higher rate of worsening of glaucoma than previously realized and that this rate may increase. However, there may be some cases in which the measurements improve.

The diagnostic ability of both perimeters was examined in receiver operating characteristic analysis (Figure 6). The highest AUC (0.911) was observed in MD with the imo perimeter (95% CI: 0.867 to 0.955). All MD, PSD, and VFI values exceeded 0.8 for both the imo and HFA perimeters, and the diagnostic abilities of the two perimeters were all significant (*P*<0.001). Moreover, the AUC of the MD was significantly higher for the imo perimeter than for the HFA perimeter.

In addition to the head-mounted configuration, other advantages of the imo perimeter are its light weight and small size, which facilitate easy handling. These features not only allow patients to be examined in bed but also expand the range of clinical applications, including the conducting of examinations in a small space[16-19].

The National Aeronautics and Space Administration is studying and elucidating symptoms of space flight–associated neuro-ocular syndrome (SANS), which occur in the whole body, nerves, and eyes during long space flights. Symptoms such as optic disc edema, globe flattening, choroidal and retinal folds, hyperopic refractive error shifts, and infarcts in nerve fiber layers have been reported to occur during long-term residence in a space station[20-21]. The imo perimeter will be a useful apparatus for performing visual field examinations in a space station.

ACKNOWLEDGEMENTS

Conflicts of Interest: **Nakai Y,** None; **Bessho K,** None; **Shono Y,** None; **Taoka K,** None; **Nakai Y,** None.

REFERENCES

1 Kimura T, Matsumoto C, Nomoto H. Comparison of head-mounted perimeter (imo®) and Humphrey Field Analyzer. *Clin Ophthalmol* 2019;13:501-513.

2 Goukon H, Hirasawa K, Kasahara M, Matsumura K, Shoji N. Comparison of Humphrey Field Analyzer and imo visual field test results in patients with glaucoma and pseudo-fixation loss. *PLoS One* 2019;14(11):e0224711.

3 Matsumoto C. New visual field examination. *J Jpn Ophthalmol Assoc* 2017;88:452-457.

4 Goseki T, Inoue T, Ookubo S. Latest equipment, Head-mounted perimeter imo. *Neuro Ophthalmol Jpn* 2017;34:73-80.

5 Matsumoto C, Yamao S, Nomoto H, Takada S, Okuyama S, Kimura S, Yamanaka K, Aihara M, Shimomura Y. Visual field testing with head-mounted perimeter 'imo'. *PLoS One* 2016;11(8):e0161974.

6 Goseki T, Ishikawa H, Shoji N. Bilateral concurrent eye examination with a head-mounted perimeter for diagnosing functional visual loss. *Neuroophthalmology* 2016;40(6):281-285.

7 Atsuko K, Michiko S, Mayumi Y. Experience in using "imo" 24plus (1) and comparison with HFA. *Atarasii Ganka* 2018;35:1117-1121.

8 Hiromasa S, Makoto A. Head-mounted perimeter imo®. *Ganka* 2016;58(8):869-878.

9 Totsuka K, Asakawa K, Ishikawa H, Shoji N. Evaluation of pupil fields using a newly developed perimeter in glaucoma patients. *Curr Eye Res* 2019;44(5):527-532.

10 Asakawa K, Ishikawa H. Pupil fields in a patient with early-onset

postgeniculate lesion. Graefes *Arch Clin Exp Ophthalmol* 2019;257(2):441-443.

11 Wakayama A, Matsumoto C, Ayato Y, Shimomura Y. Comparison of monocular sensitivities measured with and without occlusion using the head-mounted perimeter imo. *PLoS One* 2019;14(1):e0210691.

12 King AJ, Taguri A, Wadood AC, Azuara-Blanco A. Comparison of two fast strategies, SITA Fast and TOP, for the assessment of visual fields in glaucoma patients. *Graefes Arch Clin Exp Ophthalmol* 2002;240(6):481-487.

13 Udagawa S, Ohkubo S, Higashide T, Iwase A, Matsumoto C, Sugiyama K. Comparison of the glaucoma diagnostic capability and other parameters of KOWA AP-7000TM and Humphrey Field Analyzer. *J Jap Ophthalmol Soc* 2017;121:915-922.

14 Khoury JM, Donahue SP, Lavin PJ, Tsai JC. Comparison of 24-2 and 30-2 perimetry in glaucomatous and nonglaucomatous optic neuropathies. *J Neuroophthalmol* 1999;19(2):100-108.

15 Baba K, Akaike N, Harasawa K, Endo N. Practical Perimetry using Program 24-2 threshold test of Humphrey Field Analyzer. *JAPANESE ORTHOPTIC J* 1991;19:87-94.

16 Asakawa K Totsuka K, Manabe Y, Ishibe Y, Ishikawa H. Measurement of Pupil Fields in Patients with poor subjective responses. *Nihon Ganka Gakkai Zasshi* 2019;123(4):977-980

17 Asakawa K, Shoji N. Challenges to detect glaucomatous visual field loss with pupil perimetry. *Clin Ophthalmol* 2019;13:1621-1625.

18 Asakawa K, Matsuno M, Ishikawa H, Shoji N. Pupil fields in patients with Leber hereditary optic neuropathy. *Graefes Arch Clin Exp Ophthalmol* 2021;259(3):791-793.

19 Yamao S, Matsumoto C, Nomoto H, Numata T, Eura M, Yamashita M, Hashimoto S, Okuyama S, Kimura S, Yamanaka K, Chiba Y, Aihara M, Shimomura Y. Effects of head tilt on visual field testing with a head-mounted perimeter imo. *PLoS One* 2017;12(9):e0185240. DOI:10.1371/journal.pone.0185240.

20 Lee AG, Mader TH, Gibson CR, Tarver W. Space flight-associated neuro-ocular syndrome. *JAMA Ophthalmol* 2017;135(9):992-994.

21 Katura H. Space flight-associated neuro-ocular syndrome. *J Jpn Opthalmol Assoc* 2018;89:1560-1561.

Table of Contents

.

www.ingramcontent.com/pod-product-compliance
Lightning Source LLC
Chambersburg PA
CBHW040130270326
41928CB00001B/22